Keto Diet Cookbook for Beginners:

The Complete Guide to Ketogenic Diet with 28-Day Meal Plan to Lose Weight

By
Kym Coleman

The information in the following pages is broadly considered a truthful and accurate account of facts and as such, any inattention, use, or misuse of the information in question by the reader will render any resulting actions solely under their purview. There are no scenarios in which the publisher or the original author of this work can be in any fashion deemed liable for any hardship or damages that may befall them after undertaking information described herein.

Additionally, the information in the following pages is intended only for informational purposes and should thus be thought of as universal. As befitting its nature, it is presented without assurance regarding its prolonged validity or interim quality. Trademarks that are mentioned are done without written consent and can in no way be considered an endorsement from the trademark holder.

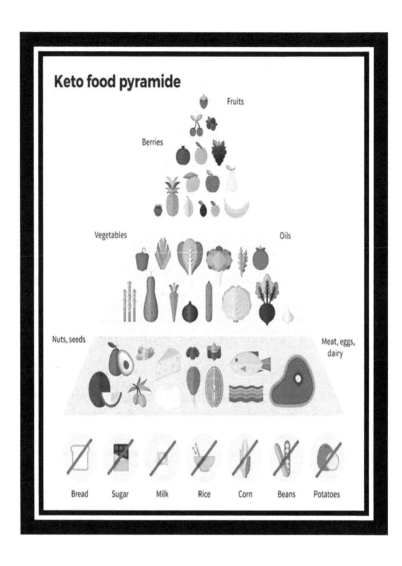

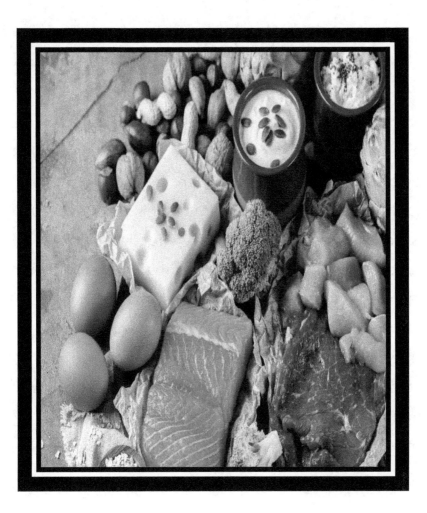

Introduction:

Did you know you can lose weight when you eat fat instead of carbs? If that sounds crazy, then you probably have not heard about the Ketogenic Diet yet. This might sound like another fad, but the truth is this diet is over 80 years old and is proven to be highly effective! In this book, you will learn the basic rules of the Ketogenic Diet, find answers to commonly asked questions about it, and most importantly, gain access to 7-day meal plans and fifty easy, delicious, and nutritious Keto-friendly recipes. To find out find out more about the Ketogenic Diet, turn to chapter one right now. Because the sooner you start making the change, the sooner you can reach your goal weight.

Chapter 1: The Ketogenic Diet

It might sound completely insane to start a diet that is rich in fat, moderate in protein, and low in carbs in order to lose weight, but science has proven this to be highly effective. Of course, this does not mean you can indulge in oily foods and animal proteins all the time, because there are several highly important guidelines to strictly follow to avoid gaining even more weight or, worse, developing a cardiovascular disease while on the Keto diet. In this chapter, you will learn the basics of the Keto diet and how it works. You will also get to know the rules to follow to safely and efficiently lose weight with the Keto diet.

What is the Keto Diet?

The Ketogenic diet is the ultimate low carb, moderate protein, and high fat diet for weight loss. However, it was not originally designed to be so. Over eight decades ago, it was used as a mainstream of therapy to help treat epilepsy in children, but it was soon discovered that it conditions the body to burn fat instead of carbohydrates for energy.

Therefore, those follow the Keto diet end up losing a significant amount of excess weight compared to those who eat high fat and high carb foods. In addition, the Keto diet shows promising results in reducing the risk of the development of neurological disorders such as Alzheimer's disease and Parkinson's disease. While the specific reason for this is yet to be discovered in detail, the overall explanation shows that the central nervous system thrives in a diet that causes the body to use fat – not glucose – as its main energy source. It is important to note, however, that weight loss and the other health benefits of the Keto diet would only take place once the body has transitioned from being glucose-dependent to being Keto-adapted – an effect that requires a minimum of 15 days of strictly following the Keto diet. Once you have become keto-adapted, you should stick to the Keto diet for the rest of their life. Otherwise, going back to a diet rich in carbs and fat will cause you to go back to being dependent on glucose, thus resulting to weight gain.

The Rules to Follow

You should only start the Keto diet if your doctor or a licensed dietitian approves it. This is because not everyone is qualified to start the keto diet, especially if they have an existing medical condition or is taking prescription medication. Therefore, you should first get professional advice before attempting this diet. Now, aside from getting your doctor or dietitian's approval, you should also be ready to commit to the rules of the Keto diet. Any deviance from the rules will instantly disrupt your path towards becoming keto-adapted. So, to set your expectations, you should be prepared to commit to the following rules for the rest of your life:

Rule#1: *You must completely avoid foods rich in carbohydrates, especially grains and sugar.*

It is important to eliminate all rich sources of carbohydrates from your diet, especially if you are still on your way to becoming keto-adapted. Your body is considered to be "keto-adapted" once it starts to rely on fat as its main source of energy instead of glucose. This can only happen if the body is sufficiently deprived of carbs, because if there is enough carbs to break down to glucose and, in turn, convert to glycogen, your body would not have to resort to burning fat. Once you have become keto-adapted and at the same time achieved the ideal healthy weight loss for your body type, you can slowly re-introduce healthy carbohydrates into your diet. However, it should amount to no more than 1 gram of carbohydrates per kilogram of your body weight. For instance, if you have reached your ideal body weight of 50 kilograms, then you should eat no more than 50 grams of carbs per day.

Rule #2: You should only choose to eat the best quality sources of natural fats.

The Keto diet promotes fat, but not just any kind of fat. Rather, it promotes the consumption of healthy fats, including those found in organic meat (grass-fed beef, free range pork, and wild game) and eggs, wild-caught fish and other seafood, organic dairy and cheese, dark chocolate, avocados, coconut and olive oils, yogurts, nuts, and seeds. You must be prepared to allocate your food budget to these sources of fats, because low quality sources can put you at risk of developing heart disease. If you think you cannot sustainably purchase premium natural sources of healthy fats, then you are not likely to sustain the Keto diet for the rest of your life and should therefore consider other more cost-effective and healthy weight loss options, such as vegetarianism or veganism.

Rule #3: You must completely eliminate trans fat from your diet.

If there is one type of fat you need to avoid regardless of whether you are on the Keto diet or not, it is trans fat. Otherwise referred to as "trans fatty acids," trans fat is the main cause of increased LDL cholesterol levels, which in turn leads to the heightened risk of heart attacks and other cardiovascular diseases. Trans fat is found in most industrially produced fats and oils, such as margarine and vegetable oil. Common examples of foods high in trans fat are baked goods such as cakes, cookies, crackers, pizza crusts, and pie crusts; packaged snacks such as corn chips, potato chips, and microwaveable popcorn; and deep-fried food, such as French fries, fried chicken, and donuts. Aside from following these three main rules in the Keto diet, it is also important for you to exercise regularly in order to allow your body to burn your excess fat stores. The more energy your body expends every day, the faster you will become keto-adapted. To help you get started on the Keto diet, turn to the next chapter to learn more about how to plan Keto-friendly meals. Also, if you have other questions regarding the Keto diet, you may find the answers to them in Chapter 3.

Chapter 2: The ideal 7-Day Keto Diet Plan

The purpose of a meal plan is more than just to ensure you are sticking to the rules of the Keto diet, for it is also meant to help you control your food budget and develop the right eating habits. It might take you some time to get used to preparing a meal plan once a week or – at the very least – twice a month, but once you do, you will realize how much easier your life is. To help you get started on the Keto diet, we have devised four ideal 7-day meal plans for you using the recipes found in the succeeding chapters of this book. Notice that the meal plans call for the same types of dishes every other day. The reason for this is to help minimize the cost and time you need to prepare your Keto-friendly meals. In other words, each recipe that calls for 4 servings, for example, literally means you will be preparing up to four meals. By doing this, you would only have to cook once for four days' worth of dinners, thus minimizing the effort you need to put into preparing your meals. With all these in mind, you should not keep food for more than 3 days inside the refrigerator and you must never reheat the food more than once. Therefore, if you are cooking for yourself, then you can halve the recipe measurements, if you like, so that you can only cook one meal for immediate serving, and another for reheating the following day or two days from the time you cooked it. Lastly, notice that the meal plans recommend at least 5 meals: breakfast, morning snack, lunch, afternoon snack, dinner, and the optional dessert. This is because eating five meals a day will prevent you from getting unhealthy cravings for the high-carb food your body was used to before you started the Keto diet. The idea is to be one step ahead of your cravings by having carefully prepared food ready and by sticking to a solid meal schedule. Try to have eat every 3 to 4 hours throughout your waking day. For instance, if you tend to wake up at 7 in the morning, then you should have breakfast on or before 7:30. Then, at 10:30 am, you should have your morning snack. At 1:30 pm, you can have your lunch. After that, 4:30 pm is your afternoon snack time. Dinner should be ready by 7:30 pm, followed by a dessert, if you wish.

All in all, you need to remember the following guidelines when it comes to planning meals for the Keto diet:

- Plan your meals ahead, at least once a week.

- Cook in bulk to save time, energy, and money.
- Store prepared meals up to 3 days in the refrigerator; reheat only once.
- Eat five small meals per day.
- Maintain fixed meal times with each meal spaced 3 to 4 hours apart.

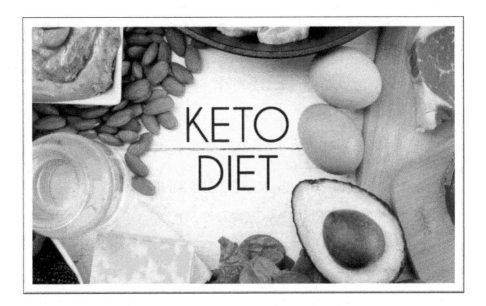

Meal Plan 1

Day 1

Breakfast: CREAMY SPINACH SCRAMBLE

Snack: CHEESY FRIED AVOCADO STICKS

Lunch: STIR-FRIED BEEF WITH MUSHROOMS AND BROCCOLI

Snack: CHEESY FRIED AVOCADO STICKS

Dinner: BEEF STROGANOFF

Dessert (optional): CREAMY CHOCO COCONUT CREAM

Day 2

Breakfast: KETO MINI QUICHE LORRAINE

Snack: CHEESY FRIED AVOCADO STICKS

Lunch: MAC-CAULIFLOWER 'N' CHEESE

Snack: CHEESY FRIED AVOCADO STICKS

Dinner: CHEESY CHICKEN THIGHS STUFFED WITH KALE AND BACON

Dessert (optional): STRAWBERRY COCONUT CREAM POPS

Day 3

Breakfast: CREAMY SPINACH SCRAMBLE

Snack: CHEESY CAULIFLOWER BITES

Lunch: STIR-FRIED BEEF WITH MUSHROOMS AND BROCCOLI

Snack: CHEESY CAULIFLOWER BITES

Dinner: BEEF STROGANOFF

Dessert (optional): CREAMY CHOCO COCONUT CREAM

Day 4

Breakfast: KETO MINI QUICHE LORRAINE

Snack: CHEESY CAULIFLOWER BITES

Lunch: MAC-CAULIFLOWER 'N' CHEESE

Snack: CHEESY CAULIFLOWER BITES

Dinner: CHEESY CHICKEN THIGHS STUFFED WITH KALE AND BACON

Dessert (optional): STRAWBERRY COCONUT CREAM POPS

Day 5

Breakfast: BLACKBERRY ALMOND MUFFINS

Snack: BARBEQUE TOFU FRIES

Lunch: BRAISED STUFFED PORK CHOPS IN MUSHROOM SAUCE

Snack: BARBEQUE TOFU FRIES

Dinner: PROVENCAL BEEF STEW

Dessert (optional): BUTTER DARK CHOCOLATE BROWNIES

Day 6

Breakfast: BAKED CHEESY EGG AVOCADO CUPS

Snack: BARBEQUE TOFU FRIES

Lunch: BRAISED STUFFED PORK CHOPS IN MUSHROOM

SAUCE Snack: BARBEQUE TOFU FRIES

Dinner: CHICKEN AVOCADO LETTUCE WRAPS

Dessert (optional): BUTTER PECAN BITES

Day 7

Breakfast: BLACKBERRY ALMOND MUFFINS

Snack: CAJUN TRAIL MIX

Lunch: GRILLED SEAFOOD AND AVOCADO SALAD Snack:

CAJUN TRAIL MIX

Dinner: PROVENCAL BEEF STEW

Dessert (optional): BUTTER DARK CHOCOLATE BROWNIES

Meal Plan 2

Day 1

Breakfast: BAKED CHEESY EGG AVOCADO CUPS

Snack: CAJUN TRAIL MIX

Lunch: ASIAN CHICKEN SALAD

Snack: CAJUN TRAIL MIX

Dinner: CHICKEN AVOCADO LETTUCE WRAPS

Dessert (optional): CRISPY CHOCOLATE-COATED BACON

Day 2

Breakfast: HAM AND BROCCOLI MINI QUICHE

Snack: CHEESY ARTICHOKE AND SPINACH SPREA

Lunch: GRILLED SEAFOOD AND AVOCADO SALAD

Snack: CHEESY ARTICHOKE AND SPINACH SPREAD

Dinner: HERB, SCALLION, AND MUSHROOM STUFFED LAMB CHOPS

Dessert: (optional): BUTTER PECAN BITES

Day 3

Breakfast: SUNNY SIDE UP EGGS OVER BACON-WRAPPED ASPARAGUS SPEARS

Snack: CHEESY ARTICHOKE AND SPINACH SPREAD Lunch: ASIAN CHICKEN SALAD

Snack: CHEESY ARTICHOKE AND SPINACH SPREAD Dinner: CHICKEN CHILI

Dessert (optional): CRISPY CHOCOLATE-COATED BACON

Day 4

Breakfast: HAM AND BROCCOLI MINI QUICHE

Snack: SAVORY SPINACH STUFFED MUSHROOMS

Lunch: SQUASH SPAGHETTI WITH MEATBALLS

Snack: SAVORY SPINACH STUFFED MUSHROOMS

Dinner: HERB, SCALLION, AND MUSHROOM STUFFED LAMB CHOPS

Dessert (optional): MINI RASPBERRY CREAM CHEESE BALLS

Day 5

Breakfast: SUNNY SIDE UP EGGS OVER BACON-WRAPPED ASPARAGUS SPEARS

Snack: SAVORY SPINACH STUFFED MUSHROOMS

Lunch: HERBED CREAMY CHEESE PORK CHOPS

Snack: SAVORY SPINACH STUFFED MUSHROOMS

Dinner: CHICKEN CHILI

Dessert (optional): KETO COFFEE CHOCOLATE CHIP COOKIES

Day 6

Breakfast: PUMPKIN AND CREAM CHEESE PANCAKES

Snack: SAVORY KALE CHIPS

Lunch: SQUASH SPAGHETTI WITH MEATBALLS

Snack: SAVORY KALE CHIPS

Dinner: MEDITERRANEAN SEAFOOD, SAUSAGE AND PEPPER STEW

Dessert (optional): MINI RASPBERRY CREAM CHEESE BALLS

Day 7

Breakfast: CHEDDAR CHEESE AND BROCCOLI MINI QUICHES

Snack: SAVORY KALE CHIPS

Lunch: HERBED CREAMY CHEESE PORK CHOPS

Snack: SAVORY KALE CHIPS

Dinner: THAI-INSPIRED BROILED CHICKEN SKEWERS Dessert (optional): KETO COFFEE CHOCOLATE CHIP COOKIES

Meal Plan 3

Day 1

Breakfast: PUMPKIN AND CREAM CHEESE PANCAKES Snack: SOUTHWESTERN STUFFED EGGS Lunch: ASIAN-INSPIRED TUNA WITH CAULIFLOWER RICE Snack: SOUTHWESTERN STUFFED EGGS Dinner: MEDITERRANEAN SEAFOOD, SAUSAGE AND PEPPER STEW

Dessert (optional): COCONUT LIME BUTTER BALLS

Day 2

Breakfast: CHEDDAR CHEESE AND BROCCOLI MINI QUICHES

Snack: SOUTHWESTERN STUFFED EGGS

Lunch: CLASSIC PORK STEW

Snack: SOUTHWESTERN STUFFED EGGS

Dinner: THAI-INSPIRED BROILED CHICKEN SKEWERS

Dessert (optional): KETO GINGERSNAPS

Day 3

Breakfast: CHEESY EGG AND BACON KETO MUFFINS

Snack: COCONUT BERRY SHAKE

Lunch: ASIAN-INSPIRED TUNA WITH CAULIFLOWER RICE

Snack: COCONUT BERRY SHAKE

Dinner: BEEF TACO SALAD WRAPS

Dessert (optional): COCONUT LIME BUTTER BALLS

Day 4

Breakfast: GRUYERE, GARLIC AND BASIL SCRAMBLED EGGS

Snack: COCONUT BERRY SHAKE

Lunch: CLASSIC PORK STEW

Snack: COCONUT BERRY SHAKE

Dinner: OVEN-ROASTED BUTTER GARLIC HADDOCK WITH SWISS CHARD

Dessert (optional): KETO GINGERSNAPS

Day 5

Breakfast: CHEESY EGG AND BACON KETO MUFFINS

Snack: SPICY GUACAMOLE WITH BACON BITS

Lunch: VEGGIE BEEF LASAGNA

Snack: SPICY GUACAMOLE WITH BACON BITS

Dinner: BEEF TACO SALAD WRAPS

Dessert (optional): KETO GINGERSNAPS

Day 6

Breakfast: GRUYERE, GARLIC AND BASIL SCRAMBLED EGGS

Snack: SPICY GUACAMOLE WITH BACON BITS

Lunch: STIR-FRIED BEEF WITH MUSHROOMS AND BROCCOLI

Snack: SPICY GUACAMOLE WITH BACON BITS

Dinner: OVEN-ROASTED BUTTER GARLIC HADDOCK WITH SWISS CHARD

Dessert (optional): PEANUT BUTTER AND CREAM CHEESE CHEWIES

Day 7

Breakfast: KETO MINI QUICHE LORRAINE

Snack: CHEESY FRIED AVOCADO STICKS

Lunch: VEGGIE BEEF LASAGNA

Snack: CHEESY FRIED AVOCADO STICKS

Dinner: BEEF STROGANOFF

Dessert (optional): CREAMY CHOCO COCONUT CREAM

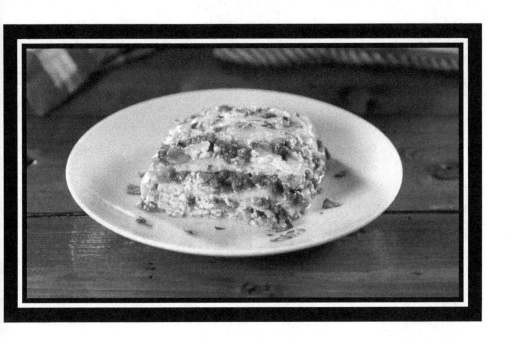

Meal Plan 4

Day 1

Breakfast: BLACKBERRY ALMOND MUFFINS

Snack: CHEESY FRIED AVOCADO STICKS

Lunch: STIR-FRIED BEEF WITH MUSHROOMS AND BROCCOLI

Snack: CHEESY FRIED AVOCADO STICKS

Dinner: CHEESY CHICKEN THIGHS STUFFED WITH KALE AND BACON

Dessert (optional): PEANUT BUTTER AND CREAM CHEESE CHEWIES

Day 2

Breakfast: KETO MINI QUICHE LORRAINE

Snack: CHEESY CAULIFLOWER BITES

Lunch: MAC-CAULIFLOWER 'N' CHEESE

Snack: CHEESY CAULIFLOWER BITES

Dinner: BEEF STROGANOFF

Dessert (optional): CREAMY CHOCO COCONUT CREAM

Day 3

Breakfast: BLACKBERRY ALMOND MUFFINS

Snack: CHEESY CAULIFLOWER BITES

Lunch: BRAISED STUFFED PORK CHOPS IN MUSHROOM SAUCE

Snack: CHEESY CAULIFLOWER BITES

Dinner: CHEESY CHICKEN THIGHS STUFFED WITH KALE AND BACON

Dessert (optional): STRAWBERRY COCONUT CREAM POPS

Day 4

Breakfast: BAKED CHEESY EGG AVOCADO CUPS

Snack: BARBEQUE TOFU FRIES

Lunch: MAC-CAULIFLOWER 'N' CHEESE

Snack: BARBEQUE TOFU FRIES

Dinner: PROVENCAL BEEF STEW

Dessert (optional): BUTTER DARK CHOCOLATE BROWNIES

Day 5

Breakfast: HAM AND BROCCOLI MINI QUICHE

Snack: BARBEQUE TOFU FRIES

Lunch: BRAISED STUFFED PORK CHOPS IN MUSHROOM SAUCE

Snack: BARBEQUE TOFU FRIES

Dinner: CHICKEN AVOCADO LETTUCE WRAPS

Dessert (optional): STRAWBERRY
COCONUT CREAM POPS

Day 6

Breakfast: BAKED CHEESY EGG AVOCADO CUPS

Snack: CAJUN TRAIL MIX

Lunch: GRILLED SEAFOOD AND AVOCADO SALAD

Snack: CAJAN TRAIL MIX

Dinner: PROVENCAL BEEF STEW

Dessert (optional): BUTTER DARK CHOCOLATE BROWNIES

Day 7

Breakfast: HAM AND BROCCOLI MINI QUICHE

Snack: CAJUN TRAIL MIX

Lunch: ASIAN CHICKEN SALAD

Snack: CAJUN TRAIL MIX

Dinner: CHICKEN AVOCADO LETTUCE WRAPS

Dessert (optional): BUTTER PECAN BITES Download the

Chapter 3: Frequently Asked questions

Q: How does the Keto diet cause you to lose weight?

A: Maintaining the Keto diet for at least 14 days will cause your liver to produce ketones, an organic compound that causes your body to start burning fat for energy instead of glucose, or the basic form of carbohydrates in the body. However, it is important to note that eating Keto-friendly meals alone will cause you to lose weight. You must remember to avoid all carbohydrate-rich foods and to start exercising regularly to boost your metabolism as well.

Q: Will going on the Keto diet increase my risk of getting a heart attack?

A: Saturated fatty acids in animal fats have been receiving a lot of flak as they are said to be linked to heart disease. However, an increasing amount of research reveals that trans fat – not saturated fatty acids – are directly linked to cardiovascular diseases. Trans fats are found in processed food such as margarine spreads and vegetable oils, therefore they should be eliminated. The rule of thumb is to avoid all processed, unnatural fats (especially those with the word "hydrogenated" found in their ingredients list) and to focus on eating the ones found in nature, such as fats from grass-fed, pasture-raised beef, organic pork, chicken, and eggs, wild-caught seafood, and of course, nuts and seeds.

Q: What makes the Keto diet more effective than other weight loss diets?

A: The Keto diet is extremely low in carbohydrates, and since excessive carb consumption – not fat consumption – is the cause of obesity, significantly reducing carbs will naturally lead to weight loss. Another reason why the Keto diet can help one lose weight more effectively is that it does not support food deprivation. People who go on extremely calorie diets often up binge-eating afterwards. However, those who are on a sustainable Keto diet continue to lose weight without losing muscle mass and without ending up binge eating.

Q: Do I need a licensed dietitian's approval to start the Keto diet?

A: Yes, you definitely need the guidance and support of a licensed dietitian before you start any kind of weight loss program. The Keto diet, in particular, requires you to monitor and measure your ketone levels at least once a week until you become keto-adapted. In addition, not all people are candidates for the Keto diet. If you have a specific medical condition such as type 2 diabetes or atherosclerosis, or if you are currently on prescription medication, you absolutely must consult a doctor before you try any Keto-friendly meals.

Q: Isn't a diet high in fat, like the Keto diet, dangerous to health?

A: A diet high in fat is only potentially life-threatening if it is also high in carbohydrates. This is because the body will still continue to rely on the glucose from the carb-filled foods for energy and any fat consumed is stored. This would naturally elevate one's bad cholesterol levels, leading to the development of atherosclerosis and other heart diseases. However, the Keto diet is high in fat but extremely low in carbohydrates. So; by significantly reduce carbohydrates from your diet and replace it instead with fat, your body will adapt to this change by resorting to fat as its source of energy.

Q: Can a person on the Keto diet have a carbohydrate "cheat day?"

A: The simple answer is No. While there is such a thing as "cyclic ketogenic dieting," or following the keto diet strictly for 5 days and then eating regular carb-filled meals for 2 days, studies note that those who apply this tend to lose lean muscle mass, which you definitely do not want to happen. Moreover, you will end up gaining even more weight if you eat carb-filled food soon after following the keto diet, because your body has not entered the ketosis yet when you start reintroducing carbs into it. The better thing to do would be to stick to a strict keto diet for at least 21 days, then very slowly reintroduce small amounts of carbs every day, or about 1 gram of carbs per kilogram of your keto-adapted body weight.

Q: Do I have to count calories when on the Keto diet?

A: In a perfect world, people count the calories they consume every day in order to ensure that they are not going beyond their daily requirements. However, in reality people have roughly different requirements depending on how they would expend their energy that day. In addition, specific issues such as endocrine or metabolic disorders have a tremendous effect on a person's daily caloric needs. It is therefore wiser to focus on eating healthy and to exercise regularly than to strictly monitor the amount of calories you consume. In the Keto diet, you should be mindful of your food choices so that you can ensure you are only eating high fat, moderate protein, and low or no carb meals every time. It is also important not to overeat even if the food is Keto-friendly, because you still need to eat less than what your body requires so that it would resort to burning its excess fat stores.

Q: Is it possible to over-consume fat in the Keto diet?

A: While eating fat and protein will make you feel satiated for a longer period of time than carbs, it is still important to remember that fat contains 9 calories per gram versus 4 calories per gram in protein or carbs. Therefore, it is definitely possible to overindulge in fatty food, even if you are on the Keto diet. To avoid overeating fat, you can use an online keto calculator to determine the maximum amount of fat in grams or calories you can eat per day.

Q: How do you know that you have entered Ketosis?

A: The most accurate way to tell if you have entered ketosis is by getting a urinalysis or a blood ketone meter. In the latter, you can tell that you are in light ketosis if the result shows 0.5 to 0.8 mmol/L; medium ketosis if it is 0.9 to 1.4 mmol/L; or deep ketosis if it is 1.5 to 3.0 mmol/L. It is also important to note that ketosis triggers headaches, lethargy, constipation, and the frequent urge to urinate. This is completely normal and the best ways to cope with the symptoms are by drinking plenty of water; eating low-carb, high fiber vegetables; incorporating psyllium fiber, chia seeds, and/or flax seeds into the diet; and taking a magnesium supplement.

Chapter 4: Keto Breakfast Recipes

(Include some diet plan Recipes)

In its simplest form, the Keto-friendly breakfast consists of a plateful of scrambled eggs with avocado and leafy greens, a side of crisp bacon, and a mug of black coffee or green tea. Of course, variety is key to keep meals interesting, especially when it comes to breakfast. So, whenever you are in the mood to change things up you should choose any of the following recipes for a healthy, hearty, and satisfying breakfast.

Creamy Spinach Scramble

Scrambled eggs are tasty enough on their own, but if you add some butter, cream, and plenty of spinach, it becomes heavenly. This recipe shows you how to create an easy, tasty, and extremely healthy hearty breakfast.

Number of Servings: 4

You will Need:

- 12 large organic eggs
- 1 onion, peeled and minced
- 2 cups chopped spinach
- 1 cup heavy cream
- 2 Tbsp. grass-fed butter
- Sea salt, to taste
- Freshly ground black pepper, to taste

How to Prepare:

Break the eggs into a large bowl and whisk well until frothy. Add the heavy cream with a pinch of salt and pepper. Mix again to combine. Place a frying pan over medium flame and heat through. Once hot, add the butter and swirl to coat. Stir in the onion and sauté until translucent. Add the egg mixture and scrape across the pan, tilting the pan to cook the runny sides. Continue to scramble until the eggs are cooked to a desired consistency – fluffy, light, and still slightly moist. Transfer to a serving plate and serve right away.

Nutritional Information per Serving Calories:

320 Fat: 32 g

Protein: 15 g

Carbohydrates: 3 g

Fiber: 32 g

Keto Mini Quiche Lorraine

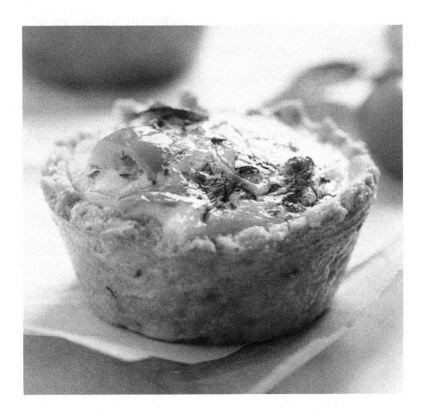

Bacon with heavy cream is best served in the morning, whether for breakfast or brunch, because they are so full of filling protein. If you want to make this recipe ahead, you should double it and use a regular pie pan instead of a mini one so that you can refrigerate the extra slices to be reheated for the rest of the week. That said, this mini quiche Lorraine is not for those who don't love cheese, because it is filled with two of the most popular cheeses on the planet: Swiss and Gruyere. Enjoy on special mornings or in mornings when you want to feel extra special.

Number of Servings: 4

You will Need:

- ½ lb. thick, organic, pasture-raised bacon strips
- 2 large organic eggs
- 2 garlic cloves, peeled and minced
- 1 large white onion, peeled and minced
- ¾ cup heavy cream
- ½ cup shredded Swiss cheese
- ¼ cup shredded Gruyere cheese
- Sea salt, to taste
- Freshly ground black pepper, to taste
- Coconut oil cooking spray, as needed

How to Prepare: Set the oven to 350 degrees F to preheat. Place the oven rack in the center section of the oven. Lightly coat a mini pie pan with the coconut oil cooking spray and set aside. Place a large frying pan over medium high flame and heat through. Once hot, add the bacon and cook for about 4 minutes per side, or until crisp and golden brown. Transfer the bacon strips on a plate lined with paper towels and set aside. Reduce the flame to medium low under the same frying pan with the bacon fat still in it. Stir in the onion and sauté until translucent for about 3 minutes. Then, add the garlic and sauté until fragrant, about 30 seconds. Transfer the onion and garlic into a bowl using a slotted spoon and set aside. Drain the bacon fat and wipe the frying pan clean. Break the eggs open into a mixing bowl and add the heavy cream. Whisk well until smooth and creamy. Fold in the Swiss and Gruyere cheeses with a pinch of salt and pepper. Then, chop the cooled bacon strips and fold them into the egg and heavy cream mixture as well, followed by the onion and garlic mixture. Mix everything well. Pour the mixture into the prepared mini pie pan. Place the pan inside the preheated oven and bake for 15 to 20 minutes, or until the quiche Lorraine is cooked through and firm. Transfer the pan to a cooling rack and let stand for about 5 minutes. Slice and serve while still warm.

Nutritional Information per Serving

Calories: 498

Fat: 42.7 g

Protein: 22.1 g

Carbohydrates: 2.3 g

Fiber: 0 g

Blackberry Almond Muffins

Breakfast muffins should not be crossed out of your list just because you are on the Keto diet. This recipe combines the succulence of blackberries and the classic taste of almonds to give you comfortingly delicious and fluffy muffins in the morning. Serve with a pat of butter or a dollop of cream cheese on top.

Number of Servings: 4 (3 muffins per serving)
You will Need:

- 2 large organic eggs
- 4 oz. fresh or frozen blackberries
- 3 cups almond flour
- 2 cups almond milk
- ¼ cup toasted unsweetened shredded coconut flakes
- 1 Tbsp. stevia 1 tsp. nutmeg
- 1 tsp. baking powder
- 1 tsp. sea salt
- Coconut oil cooking spray, as needed

How to Prepare:

Set the oven to 400 degrees F to preheat. Lightly coat 12 muffin molds with coconut oil cooking spray. Set aside. In a bowl, combine the almond flour, stevia, nutmeg, baking powder, and sea salt. Set aside. In another bowl, whisk the eggs and then add the almond milk. Mix well to combine. Gradually combine the flour mixture with the egg mixture until combined. Do not over-mix. Fold in the shredded coconut flakes and mix until thoroughly incorporated. Pour the batter into the muffin molds, then divide the blackberries among the muffin servings. Bake for 10 minutes. After that, reduce to 300 degrees F and bake again for an additional 10 minutes, or until the muffins are golden brown and puffed. Insert a toothpick into the center of one muffin; if it comes out clean, it is ready. Place the muffins on a cooling rack and let stand for 5 minutes before serving. Best served warm. Store leftover muffins in the freezer for up to 3 months; reheat before serving.

Nutritional Information per Serving

Calories: 531

Fat: 63 g

Protein: 39 g

Carbohydrates: 15 g

Fiber: 15 g

Baked Cheesy Egg Avocado Cups

Avocados are arguably the Keto crowd favorite of all the fruits, mainly because it is so rich in healthy fats! Eating an avocado half will keep you full for a much longer time than any other fruit will, plus it will nourish your body with plenty of Vitamins C and B6. Add some cheese and egg on top and you are in Keto breakfast heaven!

Number of Servings: 4

You will Need:

- 2 large avocados
- 4 organic eggs
- 6 Tbsp. shredded Colby cheese
- 1 Tbsp. freshly squeezed lemon juice
- Sea salt, to taste
- Freshly ground black pepper, to taste

How to Prepare: Set the oven to 475 degrees F to preheat. Evenly slice each avocado in half and discard the stone. Then, carefully scoop out just enough of the inside of the center of each avocado to create a "bowl" large enough for one egg. Place each avocado half, open-faced side up, into a ramekin to keep them secured. Sprinkle the freshly squeezed lemon juice over each half. Set aside. Carefully crack an egg open, separating the yolk from the whites. Slide one yolk into the prepared avocado halfand then pour its white over it. Repeat with the remaining eggs and avocado halves. Season everything lightly with salt and pepper. Top each prepared avocado and egg serving with the shredded Colby cheese. Bake for 15 minutes, or until the eggs are cooked to a desired level of consistency. Transfer to a cooling rack and let stand for about 5 minutes. Best served warm.

Nutritional Information per Serving

Calories: 324
Fat: 28.5 g
Protein: 10.8 g

Carbohydrates: 2.7 g

Fiber: 6.8 g

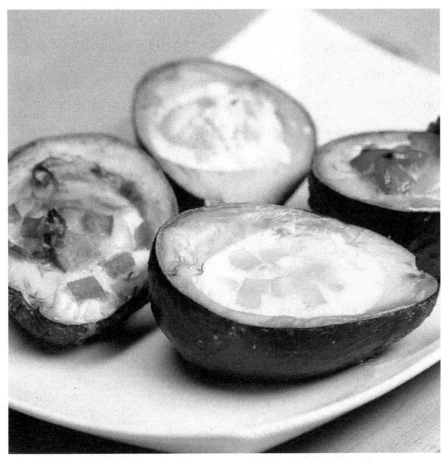

Ham and Broccoli Mini Quiche

Wake up to a healthy and filling breakfast with this Keto twist of the classic quiche. If you love the taste of this breakfast dish as much as everyone else does, you should consider doubling or even tripling the recipe. That way, you can just store them in the refrigerator for easy reheating and eating on busy mornings.

Number of Servings: 4

You will Need:
- 4 organic egg
- ¾ cup sliced organic smoked ham
- ¾ cup finely chopped broccoli florets
- ½ cup heavy cream
- ½ cup Cheddar cheese
- 1 Tbsp. olive oil
- ½ tsp. red chili flakes
- Olive oil cooking spray, as needed

How to Prepare:

Set the oven to 350 degrees F to preheat. Lightly coat a mini pie or quiche pan with the olive oil cooking spray and set aside. In a large bowl, break open the eggs and then whisk well. Pour in the heavy cream and sprinkle in the red chili flakes. Blend until thoroughly combined. Layer the sliced ham in the bottom of the pan and then layer the chopped broccoli florets on top. Sprinkle the Cheddar cheese on top of everything. Pour the egg mixture on top. Bake for 8 to 10 minutes, or until fluffy and golden brown. Transfer to a cooling rack and let stand for 5 minutes before slicing and serving. Best served warm.

Nutritional Information per Serving

Calories: 380

Fat: 28 g

Protein: 12 g

Carbohydrates: 4 g

Fiber: 6 g

Chapter 5: Keto Lunch Recipes (Include some diet plan Recipes)

Lunch Time can get really hectic, especially during the weekday. So much so that people often turn to eating fast foods and other convenient but extremely unhealthy meal options. However, it is important to stick to the Keto diet rules no matter how busy you are, so preparation and planning are key. You can make your lunch meals ahead of time easily just as long as you have a refrigerator in which to store them and a microwave in which to reheat them. Also, with the help of these lunch recipes, you will never run out of ideas on what to put into your lunchbox. Enjoy!

Stir-Fried Beef with Mushrooms and Broccoli

Lunch becomes much easier when everything you need can be cooked in one wok. This particular recipe makes use of the traditional Asian flavors of soy sauce, sesame oil, and ginger to bring out the tastiness of beef, mushrooms, and broccoli. Also, if you want to add more fiber and nutrients, you can double the amount of broccoli in each serving.

Number of Servings: 4

You will Need:

- 4 cups thinly sliced organic, grass-fed sirloin or tenderloin
- 1 large yellow onion, peeled and diced
- 1 red bell pepper, cored, seeded, and sliced into thin strips
- 2 garlic cloves, peeled and minced
- 2 cups finely sliced broccoli florets
- 2 cups chopped mushrooms
- 1 cup chopped and trimmed string beans
- ¼ cup sesame oil
- 6 Tbsp. freshly minced ginger

- 4 Tbsp. soy sauce
- 4 Tbsp. rice vinegar
- 4 Tbsp. tomato sauce

How to Prepare:

Place a large wok over high flame and heat through. Once hot, add half the sesame oil and reduce to medium low flame. Add the beef, onion, and bell pepper and stir fry until the beef is halfway cooked. Add the ginger and garlic for and sauté 30 seconds, or until fragrant. Then, stir in the broccoli, string beans, and mushrooms. Increase to high flame and stir fry for about 10 minutes, or until everything is tender. Add the soy sauce, vinegar, and tomato sauce. Mix well until the beef is cooked through and tender. Transfer to a serving platter and serve right away. Store any leftovers in an airtight container and refrigerate for up to 3 days. Reheat before serving.

Nutritional Information per Serving

Calories: 200

Fat: 22 g

Protein: 13 g

Carbohydrates: 5.5 g

Fiber: 3 g

Mac-Cauliflower 'n' Cheese

When it comes to replacing carb-filled ingredients such as pasta and pizza crusts, cauliflower is your go-to vegetable. Not only is it Keto friendly, but it is also rich in vitamins B6, C and K, riboflavin, magnesium, fiber, and protein, to name a few. If you are not fond of cauliflower, then this creamy, cheesy cauliflower mac 'n' cheese recipe will definitely change your mind and kick your pasta cravings to the curb.

Number of Servings: 4

You will Need:

- 1 small garlic clove, peeled and minced
- 2 cups chopped cauliflower florets
- ½ cup heavy cream
- ½ cup shredded Cheddar cheese
- ¼ cup shredded mozzarella cheese
- ¼ cup shredded Parmesan cheese
- 2 ½ Tbsp. cream cheese, cubed
- ½ tsp. sea salt

- Freshly ground black pepper, to taste
- Coconut oil cooking spray, as needed

How to Prepare: Set the oven to 400 degrees F to preheat. Fill a small pot with water and add half the sea salt. Stir, cover, and place over high flame. Bring to a boil. Once boiling, add the cauliflower florets and boil for 2 minutes or until fork tender. Drain the cauliflower florets thoroughly and place in a colander. Set aside to drain. Meanwhile, pour the heavy cream into a saucepan. Place over medium flame and heat through, stirring frequently. Continue to stir until the heavy cream is simmering. Stir the Cheddar and mozzarella cheeses into the saucepan, followed by the garlic. Continue to stir until melted. Turn off the heat and set aside. Transfer the cauliflower florets into a bowl and pour the cheese mixture on top of the cauliflower. Add the remaining salt and then season with black pepper. Toss well to coat. Lightly coat a baking dish with coconut oil cooking spray. Spread the cauliflower and cheese mixture in the baking dish and bake for 10 minutes, or until bubbly and golden brown. Transfer to a cooling rack and let stand for 5 minutes before serving. Best served warm.

Nutritional Information per Serving

Calories: 198

Fat: 16.8 g

Protein: 9.6 g

Carbohydrates: 2.4 g

Fiber: 0.9 g

Braised Stuffed Pork Chops in Mushroom Sauce

The braising cooking process is when you cook the meat slowly in fat within a closed pot in minimal moisture. This concentrates all the flavors from the different herbs and oils into the meat. The result is a tender masterpiece of a dish. Pack this for lunch with a side of steamed greens, broccoli, or beans. You will thank yourself later during the day.

Number of Servings: 4

You will Need:

- 4 organic, pasture-raised pork chops,
- 1 inch thick each
- 8 prosciutto slices, trimmed and chopped
- 2 garlic cloves, peeled and minced
- 1 cup mushrooms, such as porcini, trimmed and sliced
- 1 cup chicken bone broth
- ½ cup dry white wine
- 2 Tbsp. freshly grated Parmesan cheese
- 1 Tbsp. olive oil, plus more if needed
- 2 tsp. chopped fresh thyme
- 2 tsp. chopped fresh rosemary
- 2 tsp. almond flour
- Sea salt, to taste
- Freshly ground black pepper, to taste

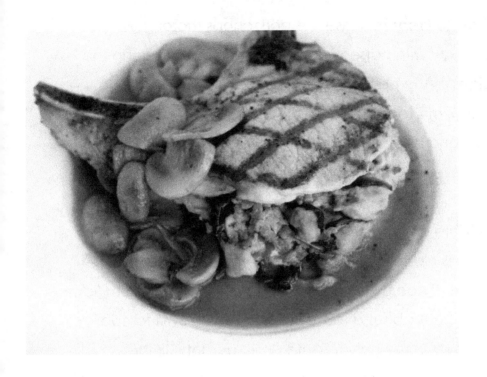

How to Prepare: Rinse the pork chops thoroughly then blot dry with paper towels. Create small slits along the sides of the pork chops to create pockets. Set aside. In a bowl, mix together 1 teaspoon of olive oil with a pinch of salt and pepper. Stir in the dried rosemary and thyme followed by the Parmesan cheese. Add the chopped prosciutto and mix well. Stuff the prosciutto and cheese mixture into the pockets of the pork chops. Crimp the edges closed or secure with toothpicks, if needed. Set aside. Place a heavy duty frying pan over medium flame and heat about a teaspoon of olive oil. Swirl to coat then stir in the garlic. Sauté until fragrant. Stir the mushrooms into the frying pan then cover and simmer for 5 minutes, or until the mushrooms are tender. Sprinkle in the almond flour and stir well to combine. Pour the chicken bone broth and dry white wine into the frying pan and increase to high flame. Bring to a boil. Once boiling, reduce to low flame and simmer until slightly thickened. Season the mushroom sauce to taste with salt and pepper, then cover and set aside. Place another large frying pan over medium high flame and heat the remaining olive oil. Add the pork chops and cook for 2 minutes per side, or until golden brown and cooked through. Pour the mushroom sauce over the cooked stuffed pork chops, then cover and reduce to low flame. Cook for about 20 minutes or until the pork chops are tender. Transfer the pork chops to a serving dish and spoon the mushroom sauce on top. Serve right away.

Nutritional Information per Serving

Calories: 300

Fat: 16 g

Protein: 34 g

Carbohydrates: 6 g

Fiber: 1 g

Grilled Seafood and Avocado Salad

This light salad is a satisfying lunch for any Keto dieter due to its combination of the creamy taste of avocado, the hearty succulence of tomato and bell pepper, and the zesty smoky flavor of the grilled shrimp. You can serve them right away or you can pack them for lunch at work. No need to reheat!

Number of Servings: 4

You will Need:

- 1 large or 2 small avocados
- 1 red bell pepper, cored, seeded, and chopped
- 1 large Roma tomato, chopped
- 1 small onion, peeled and chopped
- 1 ¼ lb. shrimp, peeled and deveined
- 2 ½ Tbsp. olive oil
- 1 ½ tsp. freshly squeezed lime juice
- ¾ tsp. garlic powder
- ¾ tsp. sea salt
- Freshly ground black pepper, to taste

How to Prepare:

Halve the avocado and discard the stone. Scoop out the flesh and slice into bite-sized cubes. Place in a bowl and sprinkle in the lime juice. Mix well to coat. Add the bell pepper, tomato, and onion to the avocado mixture. Season with half the salt and toss again to combine. Cover the bowl and refrigerate until ready to serve. Preheat the grill to medium high flame. Meanwhile, mix together the olive oil, garlic powder, half the salt, and a pinch of black pepper. Mix well and then add the shrimp and toss well to coat. Grill the shrimp for 2 minutes per side, or until pink, opaque, and cooked through. Transfer to a plate and set aside. To serve, divide the salad among four plates and then add the shrimp. Serve right away, or store immediately into airtight containers and refrigerate for up to 2 days.

Nutritional Information per Serving

Calories: 409

Fat: 25 g
Protein: 36 g
Carbohydrates: 10 g
Fiber: 5.1 g

Asian Chicken Salad

Packed with healthy fats and protein, this chicken salad will make your lunch break more special than it usually is. The spicy peanut dressing can be stored separately in an airtight container and stored in the refrigerator. You can add as much of it into your salad as you like.

Number of Servings: 4
You will Need:

- 4 organic, pasture-raised chicken breasts, skins removed
- 6 cups shredded Napa cabbage
- 2 cups shredded red cabbage
- ½ cup julienned red bell peppers
- ½ cup julienned carrot
- 2 Tbsp. chopped green onions
- 4 Tbsp. chopped fresh cilantro
- Sea salt, as needed For the Spicy Peanut Dressing:
- 6 Tbsp. natural unsweetened peanut butter
- 6 Tbsp. peanut oil
- 4 Tbsp. rice wine vinegar
- 2 Tbsp. soy sauce
- ½ tsp cayenne pepper

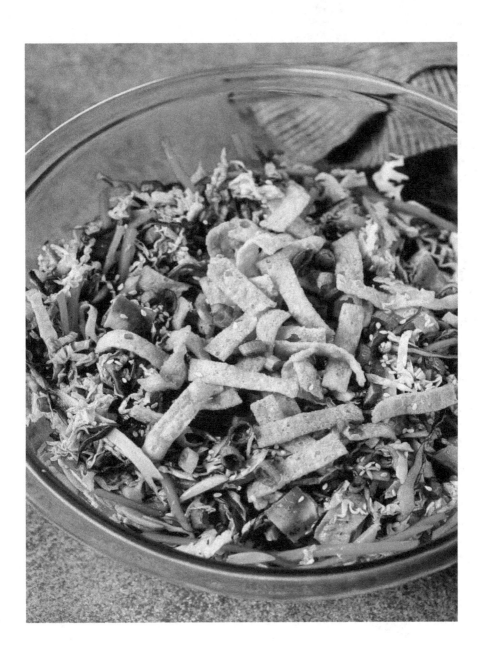

How to Prepare:

First make the dressing by combining the peanut butter, peanut oil, rice wine vinegar, and soy sauce in a bowl. Whisk well until smooth. Add the cayenne pepper and blend well to combine. Adjust seasoning, if needed. Store in the refrigerator until ready to serve. Place the chicken breasts in a saucepan and add enough water to cover. Add a pinch of salt, then cover and place over high flame and bring to a boil. Once boiling, reduce to a simmer and cook for 10 minutes, or until the chicken breasts are cooked through. Once cooked, drain the chicken breasts thoroughly and thinly slice across the grain. Place in a large mixing bowl and add the shredded cabbages, bell pepper, carrot, green onion, and about a cupful of the spicy peanut dressing. Toss well to coat. Divide the salad into four servings and top with fresh cilantro to garnish. Serve right away or store in airtight containers and refrigerate for up to 3 days.

Nutritional Information per Serving

Calories:

508 Fat: 34 g

Protein: 35 g

Carbohydrates: 12 g

Fiber: 6 g

Chapter 6: Appetizers and Snacks Recipes (Include some diet plan Recipes)

Baked Chorizo

Preparation time: 10 minutes

Cooking time: 30 minutes

Servings: 6

Ingredients:

7 oz. Spanish chorizo, sliced

1/4 cup chopped parsley

How to prepare:

Now, preheat the oven to 325 F. Line a baking dish with waxed paper. Bake the chorizo for minutes until crispy. Remove from the oven and let cool.

Arrange on a servings platter. Top each slice and parsley.

Nutrition for Total Servings:

Calories: 172

Carbs: 0.2g

Fat: 13g

Protein: 5g

Caribbean-Style Chicken Wings

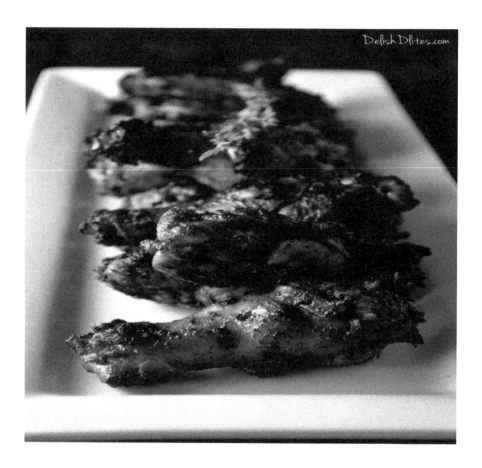

Preparation time: 10 minutes

Cooking time: 50 minutes

Servings: 2

Ingredients:

- 4 chicken wings

- 1 tbsp. coconut aminos
- 2 tbsps. rum
- 2 tbsps. butter
- 1 tbsp. onion powder
- 1 tbsp. garlic powder
- 1/2 tsp. salt
- 1/4 tsp. freshly ground black pepper
- 1/2 tsp. red pepper flakes
- 1/4 tsp. dried dill
- 2 tbsps. sesame seeds

How to prepar2:

1. Pat dry the chicken wings. Toss the chicken wings with the remaining ingredients until well coated. Arrange the chicken wings on a parchment-lined baking sheet.

2. Bake in the preheated oven at 200°F for 45 minutes until golden brown.

3. Serve with your favorite sauce for dipping. Bon appétit!

Nutrition for Total Servings:

Calories: 18.5g

Fat: 5.2g

Carbs: 15.6g

Protein: 1.9g

Rosemary Chips with Guacamole

Preparation time: 10 minutes

Cooking time: 20 minutes

Servings: 4

Ingredients:

- 1 tbsp. rosemary

- 1/4 tsp. garlic powder

- 2 avocados, pitted and scooped

- 1 tomato, chopped

- 1 tsp. salt

How to prepare:

1. Now, preheat the oven to 350 F and line a baking sheet with parchment paper. Mix, rosemary, and garlic powder evenly.

2. Spoon 6-8 teaspoons on the baking sheet creating spaces between each mound.

3. Flatten mounds. Bake for 5 minutes, cool, and remove to a plate. To make the guacamole, mash avocado, with a fork in a bowl, add in tomato and continue to mash until mostly smooth. Season with salt.

4. Serve crackers with guacamole.

Nutrition for Total Servings:

Calories: 229

Net Carbs: 2g

Fat: 20g

Protein: 10g

Golden Crisps

Preparation time: 10 minutes

Cooking time: 10 minutes

Servings: 4

Ingredients:

- 1/3 tsp. dried oregano
- 1/3 tsp. dried rosemary
- 1/2 tsp. garlic powder
- 1/3 tsp. dried basil

How to prepare:

Now, preheat the oven to 390°F. In a small bowl mix the dried oregano, rosemary, basil, and garlic powder. Set aside. Line a large baking dish with parchment paper. Sprinkle with the dry seasonings mixture and bake for 6-7 minutes. Let cool for a few minutes and enjoy.

Nutrition for Total Servings:

Calories: 296

Fat: 22.7g

Carbs: 1.8g

Protein: 22g

Spiced Jalapeno Bites with Tomato

Preparation time: 10 minutes

Cooking time: 0 minutes

Servings: 4 Ingredients:

- 1 cup turkey ham, chopped
- 1/4 jalapeno pepper, minced
- 1/4 cup mayonnaise
- 1/3 tbsp. Dijon mustard
- 4 tomatoes, sliced
- Salt and black pepper, to taste
- 1 tbsp. parsley, chopped

Directions:

In a bowl, mix the turkey ham, jalapeño pepper, mayo, mustard, salt, and pepper.   Spread out the tomato slices on four serving plates, then top each plate with a spoonful of turkey ham mixture.   Serve garnished with chopped parsley.

Nutrition for Total Servings:

Calories: 250

Fat: 14.1g

Carbos: 4.1 g

Protein: 18.9 g

Chapter 7: Keto Dinner Recipes

(Include some diet plan Recipes)

Jerk Pork

Preparation time: 15 minutes

Cooking time: 20 minutes

Servings: 6

Ingredients:

- 1/8 tsp cayenne pepper
- 1/4 tsp. salt
- 1/4 tsp. freshly ground black pepper
- 1/2 tbsp. dried thyme
- 1/2 tbsp. garlic powder
- 1/2 tbsp. ground allspice
- 1 tsp. ground cinnamon
- 1 tbsp. granulated erythritol
- 1 (1-pound/454-g) pork tenderloin, cut into 1-inch rounds
- 1/4 cup extra-virgin olive oil
- 2 tbsps. chopped fresh cilantro, for garnish
- 1/2 cup sour cream

How to prepare:

1. Combine the ingredients for the seasoning in a bowl. Stir to mix well.
2. Put the pork rounds in the bowl of seasoning mixture. Toss to coat well.
3. Pour the olive oil into a nonstick skillet, and heat over medium-high heat.
4. Arrange the pork in the singer layer in the skillet and fry for 20 minutes or until an instant-read thermometer inserted in the center of the pork registers at least 145°F (63°C). Flip the pork rounds halfway through the cooking time. You may need to work in batches to avoid overcrowding.
5. Transfer the pork rounds onto a large platter, and top with cilantro and sour cream, then serve warm.

Nutrition for Total Servings:

Calories: 289

Fat: 23.2g

Carbs: 2.8g

Protein: 17.2g

Hot Pork and Bell Pepper in Lettuce

Preparation time: 15 minutes

Cooking time: 20 minutes

Servings: 4

Ingredients:

Sauce:

- 1 tbsp. fish sauce
- 1 tbsp. rice vinegar
- 1 tbsp. almond flour
- 1 tsp. coconut aminos
- 1 tbsp. granulated erythritol
- 2 tbsps. coconut oil Pork filling:
- 2 tbsps. sesame oil, divided
- 1 pound (454 g) ground pork
- 1 tsp. fresh ginger, peeled and grated
- 1 tsp. garlic, minced
- 1 red bell pepper, deseeded and thinly sliced
- 1 scallion, white and green parts, thinly sliced
- 8 large romaine or Boston lettuce leaves

How to prepare.

1. Make the sauce: Combine the ingredients for the sauce in a bowl. Set aside until ready to use.

2. Make the pork filling: In a nonstick skillet, warm a tbsp. sesame oil over medium-high heat.

3. Add the sauté the ground pork for 8 minutes or until lightly browned, then pour the sauce over and keep cooking for 4 minutes more or until the sauce has lightly thickened.

4. Transfer the pork onto a platter and set aside until ready to use.

5. Clean the skillet with paper towels, then warm the remaining sesame oil over medium-high heat.

6. Add and sauté the ginger and garlic for 3 minutes or until fragrant.

7. Add and sauté the sliced bell pepper and scallion for an additional 5 minutes or until fork-tender.

8. Lower the heat, and move the pork back to the skillet. Stir to combine well.

9. Divide and arrange the pork filling over four lettuce leaves and serve hot.

Nutrition for Total Servings:

Calories: 385

Fat: 31.1g

Carbs: 5.8g

Protein: 20.1g

Italian Sausage, Zucchini, Eggplant, and Tomato Ratatouille

Preparation time: 15 minutes

Cooking time: 45 minutes

Servings: 4

Ingredients:

- 3 tbsps. extra-virgin olive oil
- 1 pound (454 g) Italian sausage meat (sweet or hot)
- 2 zucchini, diced
- 1 red bell pepper, diced
- 1/2 eggplant, cut into 1/2-inch cubes
- 1 tbsp. garlic, minced
- 1/2 red onion, chopped
- 1 tbsp. balsamic vinegar
- 1 (15-ounce/425-g) can low-sodium tomatoes, diced
- 1 tbsp. fresh basil, chopped
- Red pepper flakes, to taste
- 2 teaspoons chopped fresh oregano, for garnish
- Salt & freshly ground black pepper, to taste

How to prepare:

1. Add the olive oil in a stock pot, and warm over medium-high heat, then add and sauté the Italian sausage meat for 7 minutes or until lightly browned.
2. Add the zucchini, bell pepper, eggplant, garlic, and onion to the pot and sauté for 10 minutes or until tender.
3. Fold in the balsamic vinegar, tomatoes, basil, and red pepper flakes. Stir to combine well, then bring to a boil.
4. Turn down the heat to low. Simmer the mixture for 25 minutes or until the vegetables are entirely softened.
5. Sprinkle with oregano, salt, and black pepper. Stir to mix well, then serve warm.

Nutrition for Total Servings:

Calories: 431

Fat: 33.2g

Carbs: 11.8g

Protein: 21.2g

Elegant Cheese burger

Loaf Yes, this is famous!!

Ingredients:

For filling:

- 2 pounds ground beef
- 1 teaspoon salt
- About ½ teaspoon pepper powder
- 2 medium onions, finely chopped
- 2 cloves garlic, crushed
- About 4 teaspoons Worcestershire sauce For dough:
- About 3.5 teaspoons baking powder
- 2 large eggs
- 3 cups part skim mozzarella cheese, finely grated
- 3 cups very fine almond flour
- About 1.5 teaspoon xanthan gum For assembling:
- 4 tablespoons yellow mustard
- 28 slices dill pickle
- About 1 medium red onion, sliced lengthwise
- 3 cups cheddar cheese (Grated)

How to prepare:

1. Take 2 baking sheets & line them with parchment paper. Set aside.

2. To make filling: Place a large skillet over medium heat.

3. This step is important. When the skillet is heated, add beef & cook until brown. Break it simultaneously as it cooks.

4. Now remove the beef with a slotted spoon & set aside.

5. Discard most of the fat that is remaining in the skillet.

6. Place the skillet back on heat. Add onions & sauté until the onions are translucent.

7. Then add garlic & sauté until fragrant.

8. Add the browned beef & Worcestershire sauce & cook until nearly dry. Add salt & pepper & stir.

9. Now remove from heat & set aside.

10. To make dough: Add almond flour, xanthan gum & baking powder into a heatproof bowl.

11. Mix until well combined. Add mozzarella cheese.

12. Please place the bowl in a double boiler & keep stirring the mixture until the mozzarella cheese melts.

13. Remove from heat.

14. Then divide the dough into 2 equal portions. Knead the dough until well combined & soft.

15. Place one portion on each of the prepared baking sheets.

16. Shape the dough into oval shape.

17. Now place another parchment paper over the dough & roll with a rolling pin until it is of size 12 x 15 inches.

18. To assemble: Place half the filling on the middle third portion of the dough. Spread the filling lengthwise.

19. But do not spread on 1/3 portion on both the ends.

20. Then spread only in the middle third portion.

21. Fold the sides over the filling & press to seal.

22. Take a sharp knife & pierce the dough at different places for the steam to release while it bakes.

23. Now repeat the above 2 steps with the remaining dough.

24. Bake in a preheated oven at 360 to 375°F for around 25 to 30 minutes or until golden brown.

25. One thing remains to be done. When done, remove the baking sheet from the oven & let it cool properly for about 10 to 15 minutes.

26. Finally slice each into 8 pieces crosswise & serve. Try this my way!! Serves: 15 to 16

Nutrition Facts per serving:

Calories – 398.38

Fat – 31.35 g

Carbohydrates - 8 g

Protein – 24.11 g

Legendary Lemon Garlic Shrimp Pasta

I repeat... Try it if you want to. No regrets. Right!!

Ingredients:

- 4 bags Miracle noodle angel hair
- Pepper to taste
- 1 lemon, sliced
- About 1.5 teaspoon paprika
- Fresh basil to garnish
- Salt to taste
- 4 tablespoons butter
- 8 cloves garlic, crushed
- About 4.5 tablespoons olive oil
- 2 pounds large raw shrimp

How to prepare:

1. Place a large pot of water over medium high heat.

2. Bring to the boil. Drain the water in the noodles from the bag.

3. This step is important. Rinse in cold water & drain.

4. Now add to the boiling water. Boil for about 2 to 5 minutes & drain.

5. Place a large pan or wok over medium heat. When the pan is hot, add the noodles.

6. Then spread the noodles all over the pan & cook properly for a few minutes until dry.

7. Remove from heat & transfer into a bowl. Set aside.

8. Now place the pan back on heat. Add oil & butter. When butter melts, add garlic & sauté until fragrant.

9. Add shrimp & lemon slices & cook the shrimp on both the sides until it turns opaque (about 2 to 5 minutes per side).

10. One thing remains to be done. Add salt, noodles, pepper & paprika & toss well.

11. Finally garnish with fresh basil & serve.

What makes this the best? Check it out for yourself!!

Serves: 7 to 8

Nutrition Facts per serving:

Calories – 360

Fat – 21 g

Carbohydrates – 3.5 g

Protein – 36 g

Chapet 8: Keto Dessert Recies (Include some diet plan recipes)

Sugar is banned in the Keto Diet, but that does not mean you could no longer enjoy the occasional dessert. With the help of these recipes, you can recreat rich and creamy Ket-approved dessert such as ice creams and cookies at home to continue to maintain your Keto-adapted self.

Slice-and-Bake Vanilla Wafers

Preparation time: 10 minutes.

Cooking time: 15 minutes.

Servings: 2

Ingredients:

175 grams (1¾ cups) blanched almond flour

½ cup granulated erythritol-based sweetener

1 stick (½ cup) unsalted softened butter

2 tablespoon coconut flour

¼ teaspoon salt

½ teaspoon vanilla extract

How to prepare:

1. Beat the sweetener and butter using an electric mixer in a large bowl for 2 minutes until it becomes fluffy and light. Then beat in the salt, vanilla extract, coconut flour, and almond until thoroughly mixed.

2. Evenly spread the dough between two sheets of parchment or wax paper and wrap each portion into a size with a diameter of about 1½ inches. Then wrap in paper and refrigerate for 1-2 hours.

3. Heat the oven to 325°F and using parchment paper or silicone baking mats. Slice the dough into ¼-inch slicesusing a sharp knife.
4. Put the sliced dough on the baking sheets and make sure to leave a 1-inch space between wafers.Place in the oven for about 5 minutes. Slightly flatten the cookies using a flat-bottomed glass. Bake for another 8–10 minutes.

Nutrition:

Protein: 2.2g

Fat: 9.3g

Carbs: 2.5g

Calories: 101

Amaretti

Preparation time: 15 minutes.

Cooking time: 22 minutes.

Servings: 2

Ingredients:

- ½ cup of granulated erythritol-based sweetener
- 165 grams (2 cups) sliced almonds
- ¼ cup of powdered of erythritol-based sweetener
- 4 large egg whites Pinch of salt
- ½ teaspoon almond extract

How to prepare:

1. Heat the oven to 300°F and use parchment paper to line two baking sheets. Grease the parchment slightly.

2. Process the powdered sweetener, granulated sweetener, and sliced almonds in a food processor until it appears like coarse crumbs.

3. Beat the egg whites plus the salt and almond extract using an electric mixer in a large bowl until they hold soft peaks. Fold in the almond mixture so that it becomes well combined.

4. Drop a spoonful of the dough onto the prepared baking sheet and allow for a space of one inch between them. Press a sliced almond into the top of each cookie.

5. Bake in the oven for 22 minutes until the sides become brown. They will appear jelly-like when they are taken out from the oven but will begin to firm as it cools down.

Nutrition:

Fat: 8.8g

Carbs: 4.1g

Protein: 5.3g

Calories: 117

Peanut Butter Cookies for Two

Preparation time: 5 minutes.

Cooking time: 12 minutes.

Servings: 1

Ingredients:

- 1 (½) tablespoon creamy salted peanut butter
- 1 tablespoon unsalted softened butter
- 2 tablespoons granulated erythritol-based sweetener

- 2 tablespoons defatted peanut flour
- Pinch of salt
- 2 teaspoon sugarless chocolate chips
- 1/8 teaspoon baking powder

How to prepare:

1. Heat the oven to 325°F. Put a parchment paper or baking sheet with a silicone.
2. Beat in the sweetener, butter, and peanut butter using an electric mixer in a small bowl until it is thoroughly mixed.
3. Add the salt, baking powder, and peanut flour and mix until the dough clumps together. Cut the dough into two and shape each of them into a ball.
4. Position the dough ball into the coated baking sheets and flatten it into a circular shape about half an inch thick. Garnish the dough tops with a teaspoon of chocolate chips. Gently press them into the dough to make them stick.
5. Bake for 10–12 minutes until golden brown.

Nutrition:

Fat: 13.2g

Carbs: 5.7g

Protein: 4.9g

Calories: 163

Cream Cheese Cookies

Preparation time: 15 minutes.

Cooking time: 12 minutes.

Servings: 6

Ingredients:

- ¼ cup (½ stick) unsalted softened butter
- ½ cup (4 ounces) softened cream cheese
- 1 large egg, at room temperature
- ½ cup granulated erythritol-based sweetener
- 150 grams (1(½) cups) of blanched almond flour
- 1 teaspoon baking powder
- ½ teaspoon vanilla extract
- Powdered erythritol-based sweetener (for dusting)
- ¼ teaspoon salt

How to prepare:

1. Heat the oven to 350°F, and put a parchment paper or baking sheet with a silicone baking mat.
2. Beat the butter and cream cheese using an electric mixer in a large bowl until it appears smooth. Add the sweetener and keep beating. Beat in the vanilla extract and the egg.
3. Whisk in the salt, baking powder, and almond flour in a medium bowl. Add the flour mixture into the cream cheese and until well incorporated.
4. Drop tablespoons of the dough onto the coated baking sheet. Flatten the cookies.
5. Bake for 10–12 minutes. Dust with powdered sweetener when cool.

Nutrition:

Fat: 13.7g

Carbs: 3.4g

Protein: 4.1g

Calories: 154

Mocha Cream Pie

Preparation time: 15 minutes.

Cooking time: 5 minutes.

Servings: 10

Ingredients:

- 1 cup strongly brewed coffee, at room temperature
- 1 easy chocolate pie crust
- 1 cup heavy whipping cream
- 1 (½) teaspoon grass-fed gelatin
- 1 teaspoon vanilla extract
- ¼ cup cocoa powder
- ½ cup powdered erythritol-based sweetener

How to prepare:

1. Grease a 9-inch glass or ceramic pie pan. Press the crust mixture evenly and firmly to the sides of the greased pan or its bottom. Refrigerate until the filling is prepared.

2. Pour the coffee into a small saucepan and add gelatin. Whisk thoroughly and then place over medium heat. Allow it to simmer, whisking from time to time to make sure the gelatin dissolves. Allow it to cool for 20 minutes.

3. Add the vanilla extract, cocoa powder, sweetener, and cream into a large bowl. Use an electric mixer to beat until it holds stiff peaks.
4. Add the gelatin mixture that has been cooled and beat until it is well incorporated. Pour over the cooled crust and place in the refrigerator for 3 hours until it becomes firm.

Nutrition:

Fat: 20.2 g

Carbs: 6.2g

Fiber: 3.1g

Calories: 218

Coconut Custard Pie

Preparation time: 10 minutes.

Cooking time: 50 minutes.

Servings: 8

Ingredients:

- 1 cup heavy whipping cream
- ¾ cup powdered erythritol-based sweetener
- ½ cup full-fat coconut milk
- 4 large eggs

- ½ stick (¼ cup) of cooled, unsalted, melted butter
- 1 (¼) cups unsweetened shredded coconut
- 3 tablespoon coconut flour
- ½ teaspoon baking powder
- ½ teaspoon vanilla extract
- ¼ teaspoon salt

How to prepare:

1. Heat the oven to 350°F and grease a 9-inch ceramic pie pan or glass.
2. Place the melted butter, eggs, coconut milk, sweetener, and cream in a blender. Blend well.
3. Add the vanilla extract, baking powder, salt, coconut flour, and a cup of shredded coconut. Continue blending.
4. Empty the mixture into the pie pan and sprinkle with the rest of the shredded coconut. Bake for 40–50 minutes. Stop when the center moves, but the sides are set.
5. Take out of the oven and allow it to cool for 30 minutes. Place in the refrigerator and allow to stay for 2 hours before cutting it.

Nutrition:

Fat: 29.5g

Carbs: 6.7g

Protein: 5.3g

Calories: 317

Coconut Macaroons

Preparation time: 10 minutes.

Cooking time: 8 minutes.

Servings: 20–40 cookies.

Ingredients:

- 0.33 cups water
- 0.75 cups monk fruit sweetener or less to taste)
- 0.25 teaspoon sea salt
- 0.75 teaspoon sugar-free vanilla extract
- 2 eggs, large
- 3–4 cups unsweetened shredded coconut, or more as desired
- Optional: Sugar-free chocolate chips

How to prepare:

1. Set the oven setting to 350°F.
2. Lightly spray a cookie tin with a spritz of cooking oil spray.
3. In a small saucepan, pour in the water and the sweetener, salt, and vanilla extract. Bring to a boil using the med-high heat temperature setting. Stir and remove from the heat.
4. Use a food processor to combine the egg and coconut flakes. Pour in the syrup and process to form the dough. Using a cookie scoop, place mounds about an inch apart onto the cookie sheet.
5. Bake for 8 minutes, and rotate the baking pan in the oven.
6. Bake until lightly browned or for an additional four minutes.
7. Cool on a rack. Drizzle with melted chocolate to your liking.

Nutrition:

Calories: 24kcal

Protein: 0.62g

Fat: 0.55g

Carbs: 4.09g

Orange and Cranberries Cookies

Preparation time: 15 minutes.

Cooking time: 10 minutes.

Servings: 18

Ingredients:

- 0.75 cup butter—softened
- 3 eggs
- 0.5 cup coconut flour
- 1.5 teaspoon baking powder
- 0.75 cup monk fruit sweetener
- 0.25 teaspoon baking soda
- 0.25 cup sugar-free dried cranberries
- 0.5 cup macadamia nuts chopped
- 1.5 teaspoon dried grated orange zest

How to prepare:

1. In a mixing container, beat the sweetener with the eggs and butter until well combined.
2. Sift the coconut flour with the baking powder and soda. Beat on the low setting or with a spoon until fully mixed.
3. Fold in the cranberries, orange zest, and nuts.
4. Shape into rounds and arrange on the cookie sheet.

5. Arrange the cookies a minimum of one inch apart for baking on a parchment-lined cookie sheet. Press each mound down slightly to flatten.

6. Bake at 350°F until edges have started to brown or for eight to ten minutes. Cool for a few minutes,

7. Transfer to a cooling rack. Enjoy right out of the fridge for a week or they can be frozen for longer storage.

Nutrition:

Carbs: 2g

Protein: 3g

Fats: 19g

Calories: 200

COOKING CONVERSION CHART

Measurement

CUP	ONCES	MILLILITERS	TABLESPOONS
8 cup	64 oz	1895 ml	128
6 cup	48 oz	1420 ml	96
5 cup	40 oz	1180 ml	80
4 cup	32 oz	960 ml	64
2 cup	16 oz	480 ml	32
1 cup	8 oz	240 ml	16
3/4 cup	6 oz	177 ml	12
2/3 cup	5 oz	158 ml	11
1/2 cup	4 oz	118 ml	8
3/8 cup	3 oz	90 ml	6
1/3 cup	2.5 oz	79 ml	5.5
1/4 cup	2 oz	59 ml	4
1/8 cup	1 oz	30 ml	3
1/16 cup	1/2 oz	15 ml	1

Temperature

FAHRENHEIT	CELSIUS
100 °F	37 °C
150 °F	65 °C
200 °F	93 °C
250 °F	121 °C
300 °F	150 °C
325 °F	160 °C
350 °F	180 °C
375 °F	190 °C
400 °F	200 °C
425 °F	220 °C
450 °F	230 °C
500 °F	260 °C
525 °F	274 °C
550 °F	288 °C

Weight

IMPERIAL	METRIC
1/2 oz	15 g
1 oz	29 g
2 oz	57 g
3 oz	85 g
4 oz	113 g
5 oz	141 g
6 oz	170 g
8 oz	227 g
10 oz	283 g
12 oz	340 g
13 oz	369 g
14 oz	397 g
15 oz	425 g
1 lb	453 g

Conclusion:

Now that you have obtained a large collection of Keto-friendly recipes as well as four 7-day meal plans, the only thing left for you to do is to get started! So, go ahead and schedule an appointment with your doctor or licensed dietician right now. Find out more about the Keto diet and determine whether you can start it and how. Next, get rid of all the sugar and grains from your kitchen and replace them with Keto-approved ingredients. After that, you can finally create your meal plans, gather your ingredients, and start cooking! The sooner you take steps towards weight loss, the sooner you will achieve your health goals.

CPSIA information can be obtained
at www.ICGtesting.com
Printed in the USA
BVHW052014080521
606756BV00003B/584